What's in Your Mouth?

Your Guide to a Lifelong Smile

Douglas A. Terry, DDS

Editorial Assistant
Melissa Nix

Advisors
John O. Burgess, DDS, MS
Cynthia P. Trajtenberg, DDS, MS
Susana B. Paoloski, DDS
Catherine M. Flaitz, DDS, MS
Rocio Barocio, DDS
Kim S. Gee, DDS, MS

Clinical and Photographic Contributors
Deepak Mehta, BDS, MDS
Shankargouda Patil, BDS, MDS
Ashwini Santosh, BDS, MDS

quintessence books

Quintessence Publishing Co, Inc
Chicago, Berlin, Tokyo, London, Paris, Milan, Barcelona, Beijing,
Istanbul, Moscow, New Delhi, Prague, São Paulo, Seoul, Singapore, and Warsaw

I would like to express my gratitude to my dedicated team—Melissa Nix, Ernesto de Haro Tostado, and Rocio Barocio—for their relentless work ethic and continued commitment to excellence. This project would not have seen daylight without the dedication, organization, and imagination of Captain Leah Huffman, Sue Robinson, Ted Pereda, Angelina Sanchez, and Kristina Hartman from the Quintessence team. Also, a special recognition to Sue Terry, who is not only my mother but also my best friend and my most attentive critic. Most important, to my Creator who makes me realize that teeth and gums are simple in His hands but so complex in mine.

Library of Congress Cataloging-in-Publication Data
Terry, Douglas A., author.
 What's in your mouth? Your guide to a lifelong smile / Douglas A. Terry.
    pages cm
 ISBN 978-0-86715-666-9 (alk. paper)
 1. Mouth--Care and hygiene. 2. Dental hygiene. 3. Periodontal disease--Prevention. I. Title.
 RK60.7.T47 2014
 617.6'01--dc23
                          2013048963

quintessence books

© 2014 Quintessence Publishing Co Inc

Quintessence Publishing Co Inc
4350 Chandler Drive
Hanover Park, IL 60133
www.quintpub.com

5 4 3 2 1

Editor: Leah Huffman
Design: Ted Pereda
Production: Angelina Sanchez

This sequel to *What's in Your Mouth? What's in Your Child's Mouth?* was created at the request of both professionals and patients. After repeated review of the children's book, they asked for a similar guide for adults.

One of my patients of many years, Stephan, taught me the importance of making the patient the team captain for his improved oral health. In the past 14 years, I have learned from my patients that in order to ensure a lifelong smile, the patient must adopt the oral health philosophy of our dental team. Longevity of the dentition can only be achieved with proper brushing and flossing and routine maintenance visits by the patient. Patients can only improve on their maintenance regimen through continued supervision at each maintenance visit.

The inspiration for sharing my experiences in oral health management can be attributed to my dear colleagues and students around the world. They have expressed interest during presentations and hands-on demonstrations. These inquiries on soft tissue management have initiated this compilation of explanation.

The photographs in this book illustrate the ways we teach our patients like Stephan to brush and floss and the consequences of neglecting their teeth and gums. Our goal as health care providers is to inform patients of the importance of daily care, routine visits to their dentist, and oral cancer screening. Patients like Stephan realize that they can become part of the solution for longevity of the dentition and improved oral health. I hope you become part of the solution for improved oral health, minimal dental treatment, and a lifelong smile.

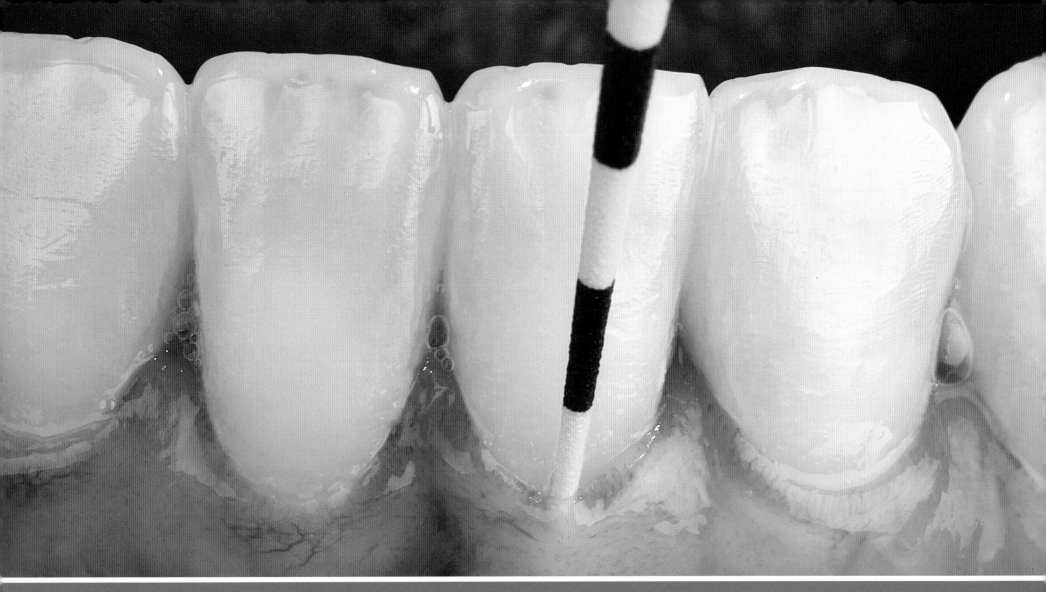

Gum disease is caused by plaque—a creamy white or yellowish film of bacteria on the surfaces of your teeth and gums. A healthy mouth is free of plaque, and healthy gums appear light pink in color with a surface texture similar to a dull orange peel. Healthy gums also do not bleed upon periodontal probing, as shown here.

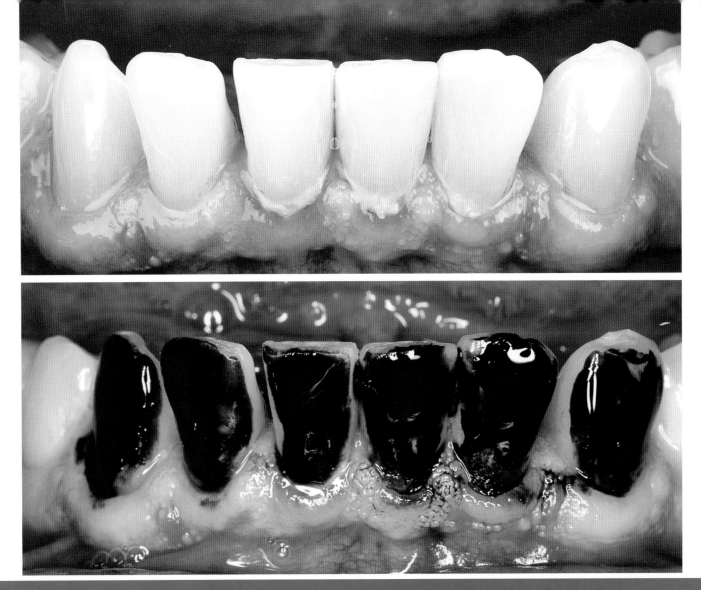

Dental plaque is a creamy white to yellow, sticky film that forms on teeth when bacteria in the mouth mix with saliva and any food left in the mouth after eating. This mixture forms an acid that can weaken the enamel and cause tooth decay and gum disease.

A plaque-disclosing agent can identify areas of your teeth that still retain plaque and that require more attention during your oral care routine. Plaque-disclosing products contain a harmless dye that reacts with the plaque, exposing it to view.

This patient thought he had successfully cleaned his teeth, but the disclosing dye revealed otherwise.

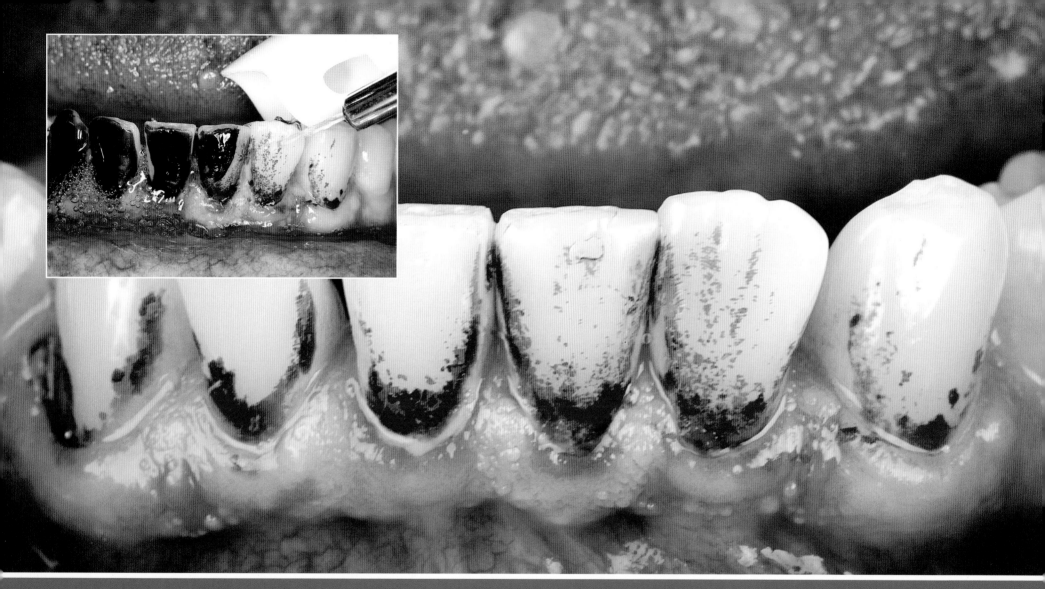

After rinsing, the remaining dyed areas identify the trouble spots that need more attention when brushing and flossing. Disclosing gel can also distinguish among fresh plaque, mature plaque, and strong acid-producing plaque with different colors. A pink or red color indicates that the plaque is new. A blue or purple color indicates that the plaque has been on the tooth for at least 48 hours. A light blue color indicates a strong acid-producing plaque that has been there even longer. Remember that plaque comes back every 24 hours, so you need to brush and floss every day.

For this patient, the gel shows that the plaque has been on his teeth for several days, increasing his risk for tooth decay and gingivitis. Now he knows which areas he needs to spend more time on while brushing and flossing.

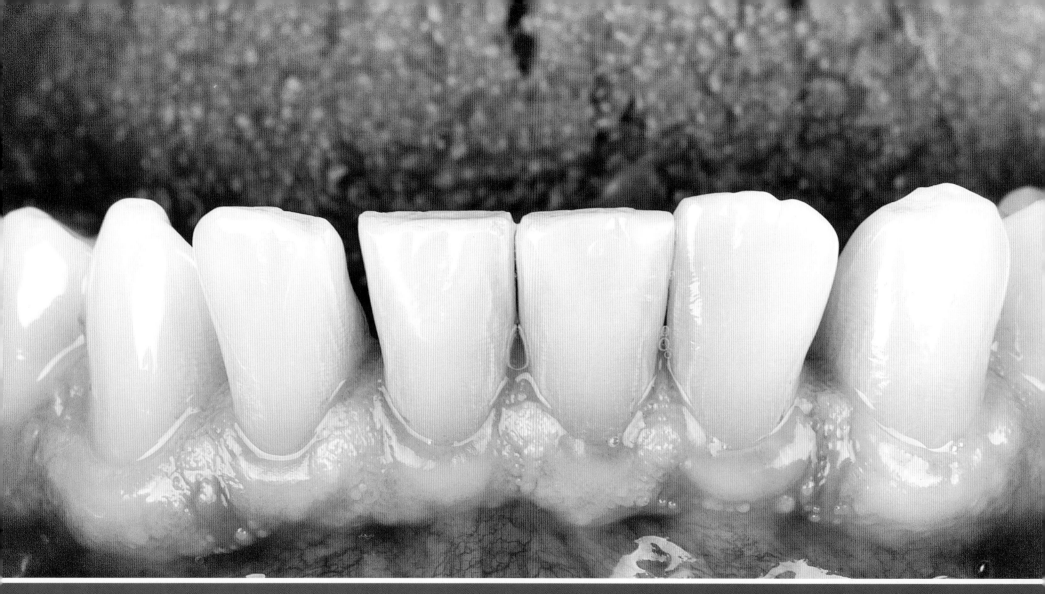

After brushing thoroughly, the plaque is removed from the teeth.

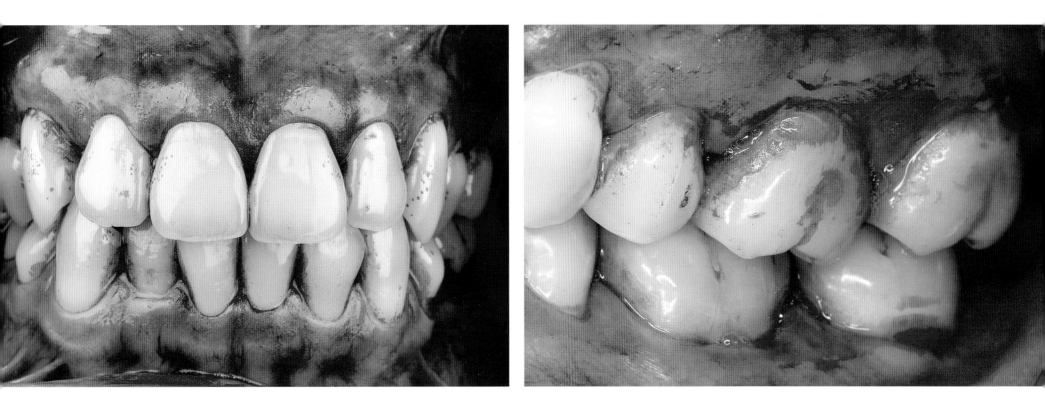

This adult patient thought she was brushing thoroughly. The disclosing agent, however, indicates that she brushes well on her front teeth but does not effectively remove the plaque on her back teeth. Also, notice that there is plaque in between the front teeth, indicating that she has not been flossing.

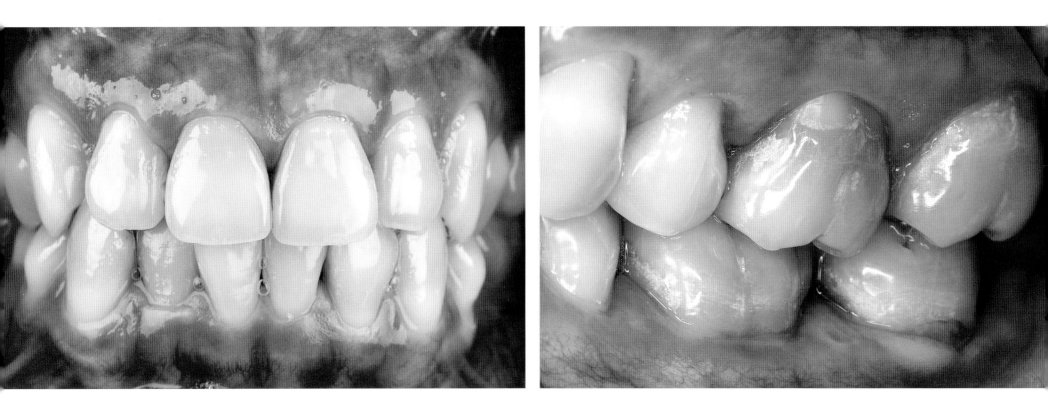

This disclosing technique allows patients to visualize the missed plaque and evaluate the effectiveness or ineffectiveness of their method of brushing and flossing. Note how clean the patient's teeth are after she improved her brushing and flossing technique, as illustrated by the minimal amount of pink dye on the teeth. However, the patient will need to return for periodic maintenance visits to remove the residual staining and calculus deposits that have accumulated as a result of her prior ineffective brushing technique.

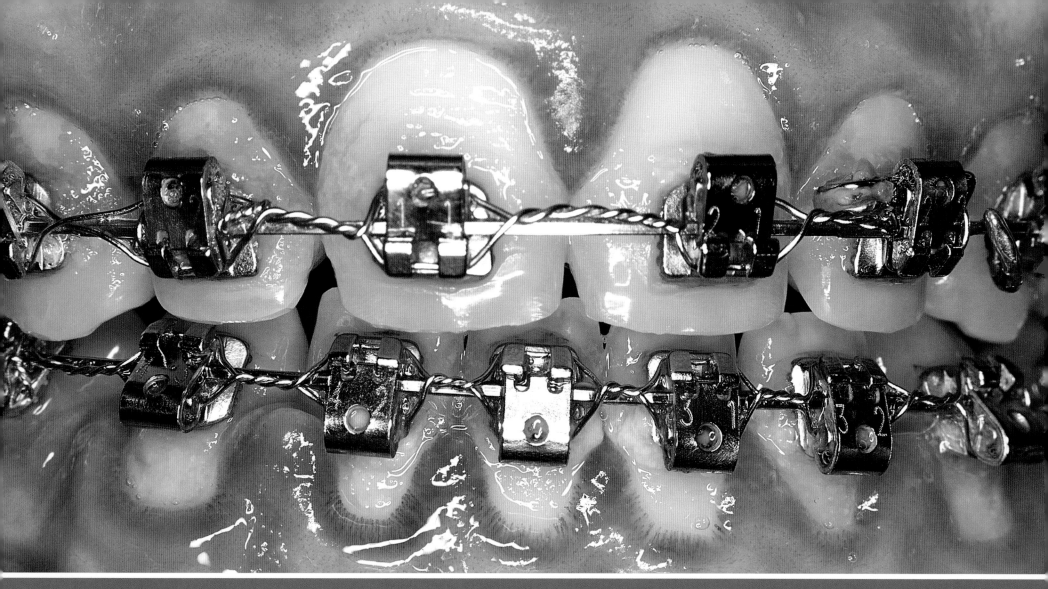

Gingivitis is a very common reversible form of gum disease that causes irritation, redness, and inflammation of the gums. The most common cause of gingivitis is poor oral hygiene.

This adult patient neglected routine brushing and flossing and left plaque on the teeth and gums, which resulted in inflammation and redness of the gums, a condition called *plaque-induced gingivitis*. Symptoms of gingivitis include swollen gums, bright red or purple gums, bleeding gums, gums that are mildly tender during brushing or painful to the touch, and bad breath.

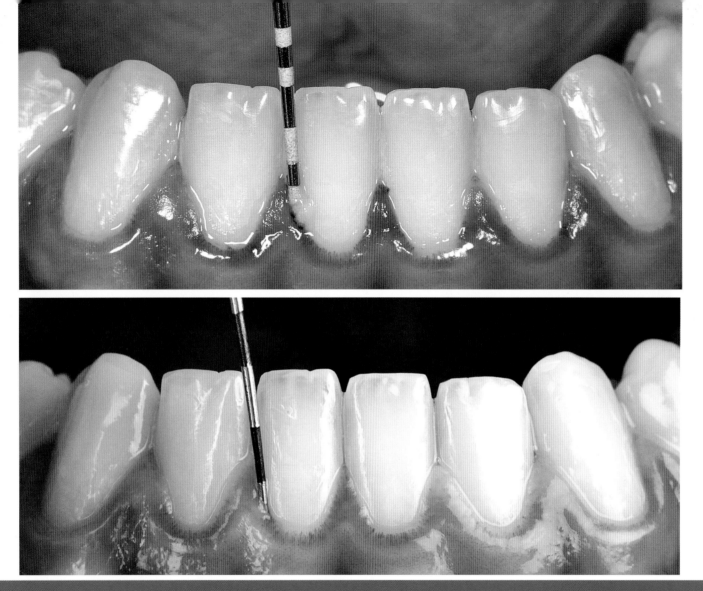

The cause of plaque-induced gingivitis is bacterial plaque. The bacteria in plaque produce enzymes and toxins that degrade tissues and promote a local inflammatory response in the gum tissue *(top photograph)*. This inflammation can also spread to distant organs in the body, such as the heart and joints.

Plaque-induced gingivitis can be prevented by eliminating the causative agent: plaque. Therapy consists of removal of plaque, which includes daily brushing and flossing and regular periodic visits to a dental professional. In addition, as part of a daily oral care regimen, the use of antiseptic rinses has been proven to be effective in preventing gingivitis. Note the improvement in the gum tissue after the elimination of plaque *(bottom photograph)*.

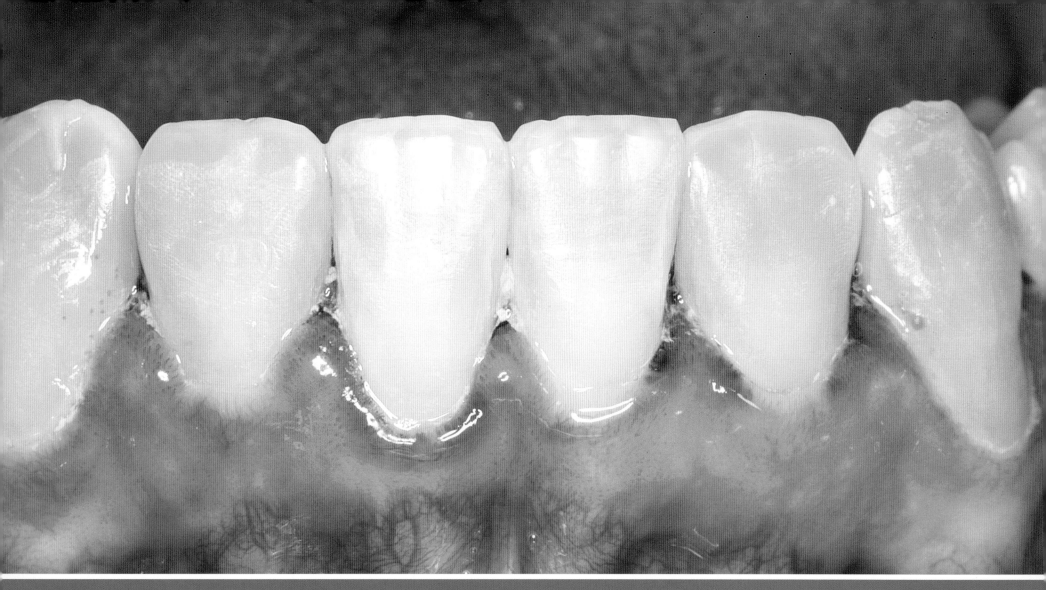

Statistics reveal that 50% to 75% of all pregnant women develop pregnancy gingivitis. During pregnancy, the elevation in hormones alters the body's response to bacteria, so the gums can become swollen and tender and can bleed upon brushing and flossing. The severity of pregnancy gingivitis usually increases during the second trimester. This condition is reversible with daily and proper oral hygiene, routine professional cleanings, and good nutrition.

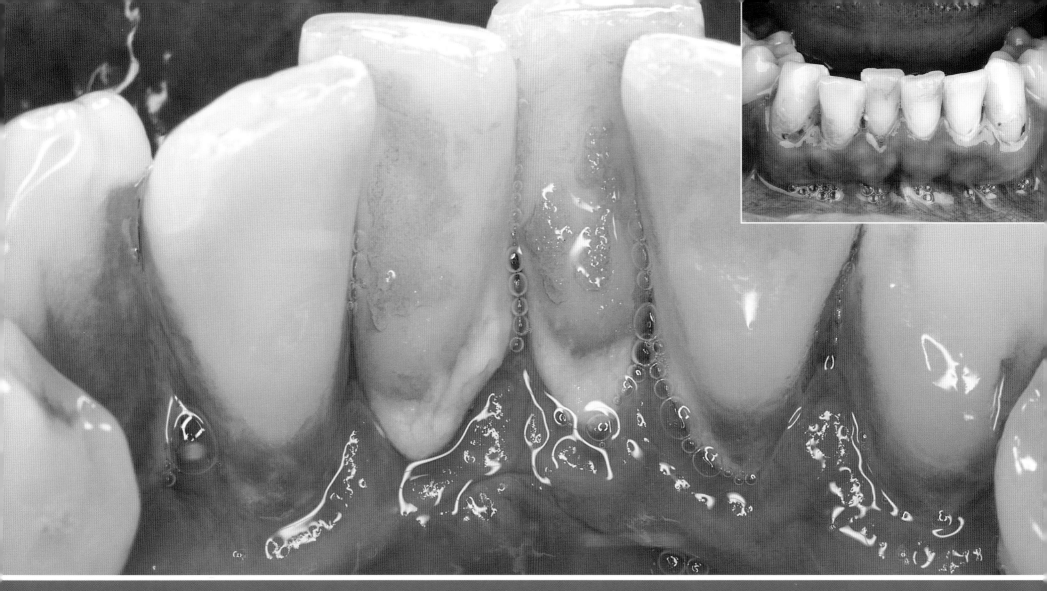

Calculus (also known as *tartar*) is mineralized plaque, and its rough layered structure provides an excellent site for further plaque growth and mineralization with calcium phosphate. There are two main types of calculus: supragingival (above the gum line) and subgingival (below the gum line). The inside surfaces of the lower teeth are near the openings of the salivary glands and exhibit supragingival calculus deposits. The outside surfaces of the lower incisors *(inset)* exhibit deposits of subgingival calculus. This subgingival calculus is usually darker in color and harder than the loosely structured supragingival calculus. Malpositioned incisors do not benefit from the cleaning action of the lower lip and tongue, so more thorough oral hygiene is required for such teeth.

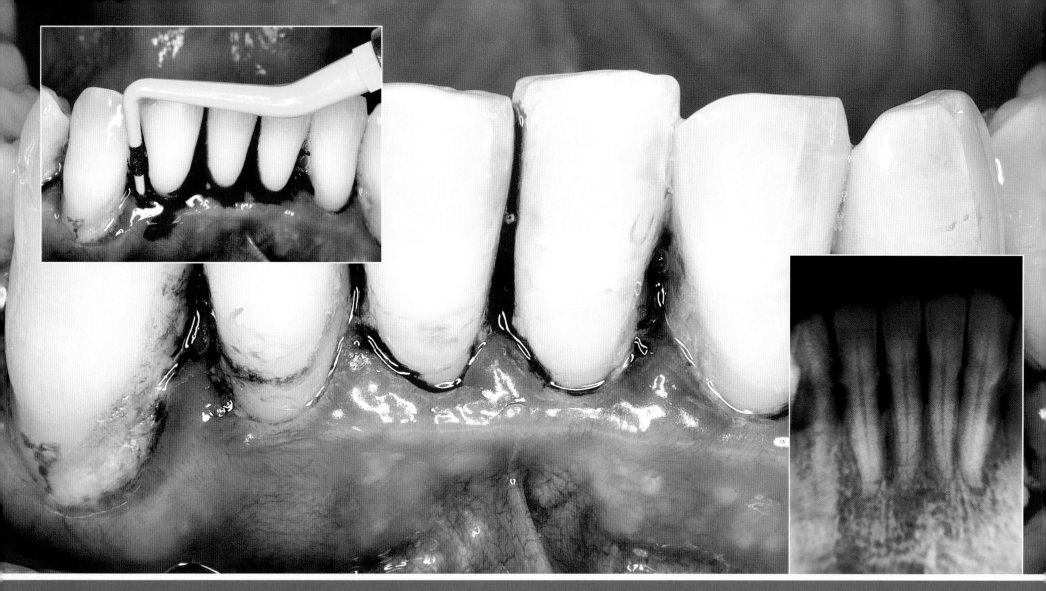

Chronic periodontitis is the most common type of periodontitis and involves progressive loss of the tooth-supporting structures (bone and gum tissues). It is caused by bacterial plaque accumulation and usually develops from preexisting untreated gingivitis. The supporting bone and tissues are destroyed by toxins produced by the bacteria in plaque, and the gums separate from the teeth, forming spaces between the teeth and gums called *pockets* that become infected. Diagnosis of periodontal disease requires a thorough medical history, periodontal examination of the gum tissues around the teeth with a probe, and x-rays to determine the amount of bone loss around the teeth. Signs and symptoms of periodontitis include red, swollen, and bleeding gums; gum recession; deep pockets around the teeth; bad breath; and moving/drifting teeth.

This patient had only mild symptoms, was diagnosed with chronic periodontitis, and was treated by a periodontist (gum specialist). Treatment required gum surgery.

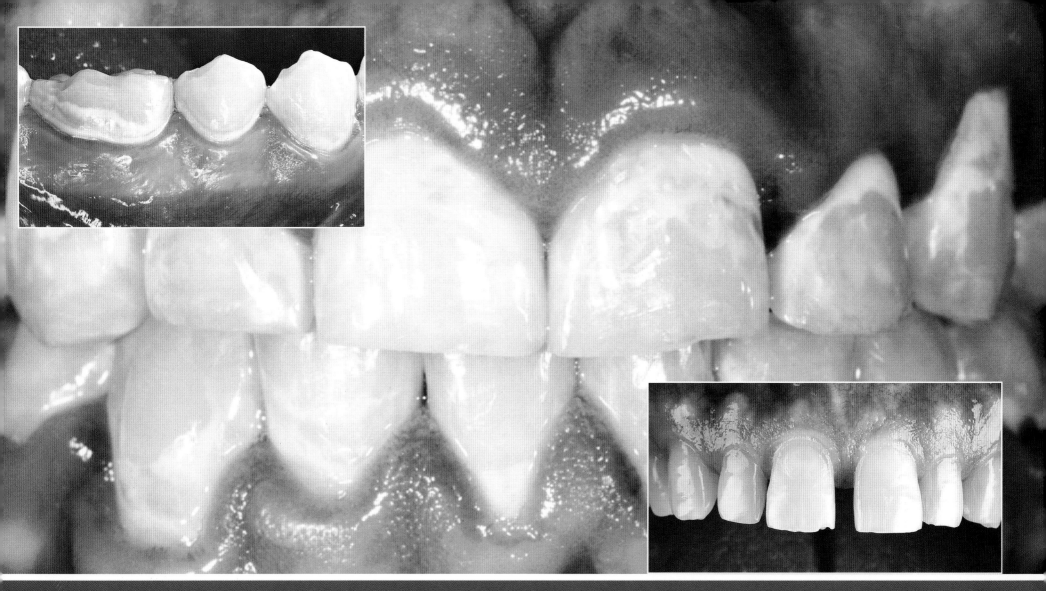

Demineralization is the process by which strong acids dissolve minerals in dental enamel. When minerals are dissolved from enamel, the tooth can become more sensitive; if there is a large depletion of minerals, the enamel can lose its structural integrity, resulting in a cavity. The acids that cause demineralization are found in foods such as tomatoes, lemons, and oranges. The patient in the photograph at right sucked on lemons, resulting in significant demineralization. Acids are also produced as byproducts of bacteria in the mouth that feed on starches and sugars (especially refined starches and sugars).

These patients left plaque on the gum line of their teeth, resulting in "white spots," an early demineralization stage for decay. Daily improved brushing and flossing with the use of toothpaste, gels, or rinses containing fluoride, alone or in combination with calcium and phosphate, can prevent this process from occurring on your teeth.

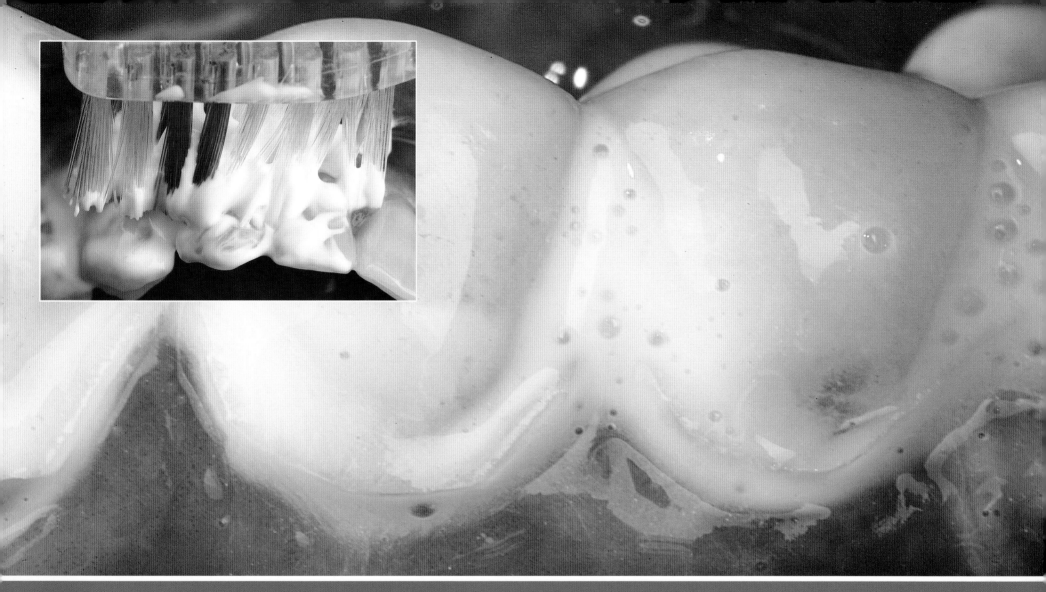

Remineralization is the process by which mineral ions are replaced in the enamel structure of the tooth. Natural remineralization occurs with minerals in our saliva taken from specific foods high in mineral content. However, conditions in the mouth such as highly acidic saliva can prevent this process. Therefore, the use of products containing fluoride alone or in combination with calcium and phosphate (such as toothpaste, gels, or mouthwash) can be used to maintain the proper acid level (pH) of your saliva, prevent demineralization, and enhance remineralization.

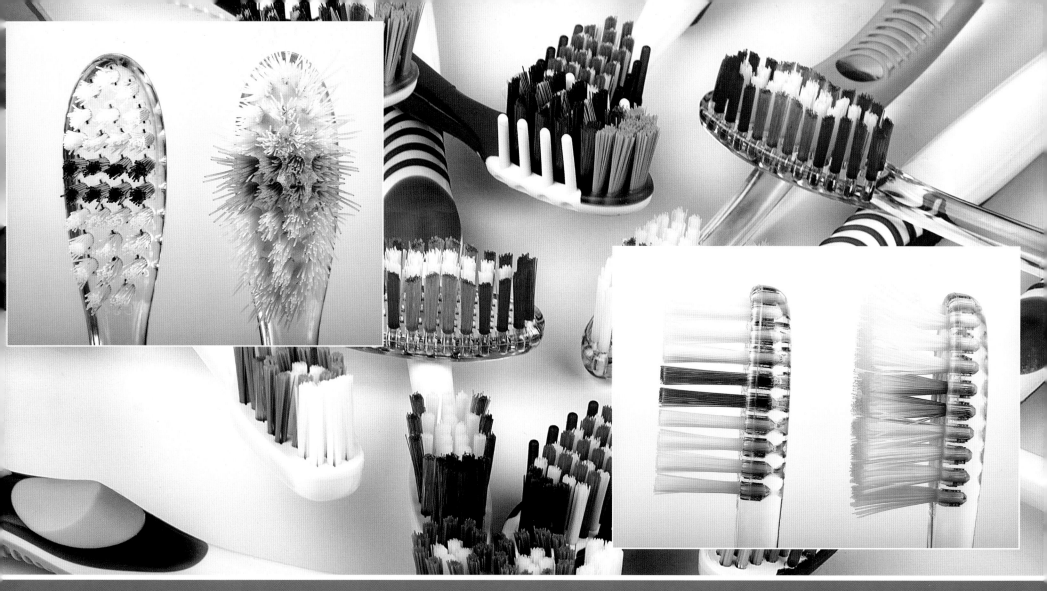

Teeth come in different shapes and sizes, and there are several different toothbrush varieties available. No matter which variety you use, toothbrush bristles can become worn and frayed over time, decreasing their effectiveness. It is important that you not share your toothbrush with anyone and that you replace your toothbrush every 2 to 3 months and whenever you have a cold or sinus infection (to prevent reinfection). Smart toothbrushes have color changes that indicate when it is time to replace the brush.

Because your toothbrush is exposed to germs, viruses, and bacteria every day, you may want to soak it in mouthwash, vinegar, or hydrogen peroxide for several hours to disinfect it. Always rinse and dry the toothbrush before reuse.

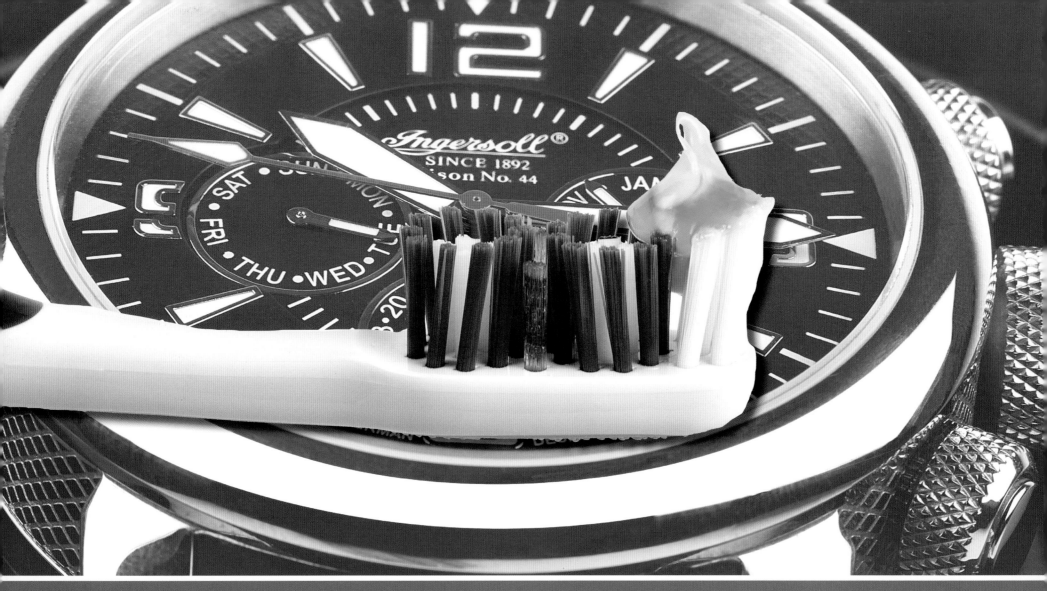

The bristles of the toothbrush, not the toothpaste, clean the teeth, but toothpaste freshens breath and strengthens teeth against bacteria. However, you only need a tiny bit of toothpaste (the size of a pea) to get the job done. Too much toothpaste can make brushing harder because of all the foam in the mouth. Effective plaque removal requires at least 2 minutes of brushing twice a day.

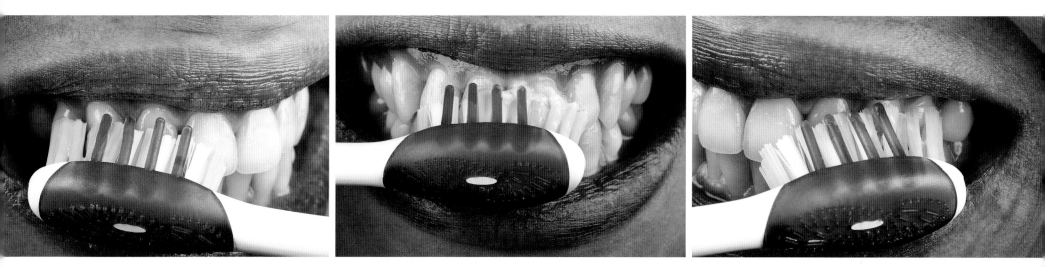

The way you brush is more important than what you brush with, so you should use the following brushing technique. On the outer and inner surfaces, place the bristles of the brush along the gum line at a 45-degree angle to the tooth. The bristles should contact both the tooth surface and the gum line using short, half-tooth-wide vibratory strokes.

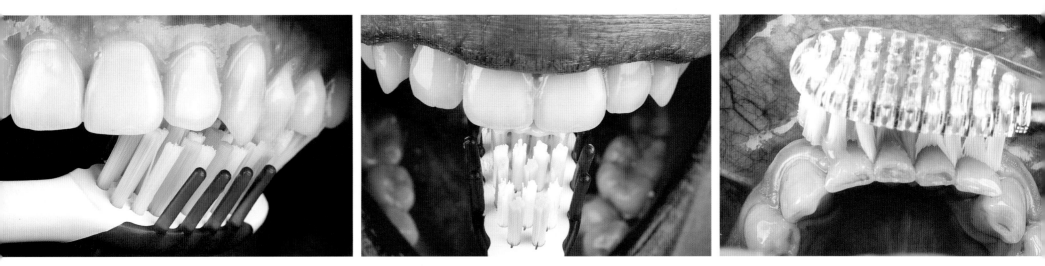

On the chewing surfaces, hold the brush flat against the biting surfaces of the teeth and brush back and forth. On the inside surfaces of front teeth, tilt the brush vertically behind the front teeth and use gentle up and down strokes using the top half of the brush. Remember to angle the brush toward the gum line when brushing the outer surfaces of your front teeth.

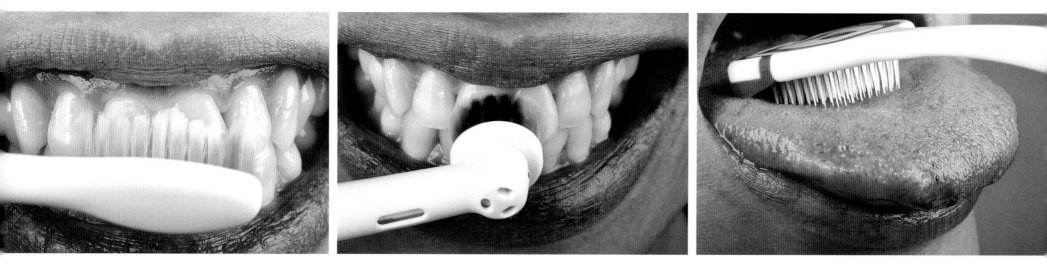

Powered toothbrushes now come in all sizes and shapes with a variety of features, such as pressure sensors and timers. There are different brushing actions for powered toothbrushes, but all powered brushes are just as safe and gentle as manual toothbrushes for the gums and teeth. Even with powered brushes, however, you should use the same technique and spend the same amount of time as you would for manual brushing and change the bristles every 2 to 3 months.

To obtain the most benefit from brushing your teeth, you should brush your tongue as well. Bacteria are present on the tongue in enormous quantities, and these bacteria can transfer to your teeth within a few hours after brushing. Research has shown that tongue cleaners are more effective than regular toothbrushes in removing debris and bacteria. Place the tongue cleaner as far back as possible and brush the tongue in a back-to-front sweeping motion. Practice is required to find the correct positioning of the brush to minimize gagging. Individuals with halitosis are advised to repeat the tongue-cleaning procedure several times during the day.

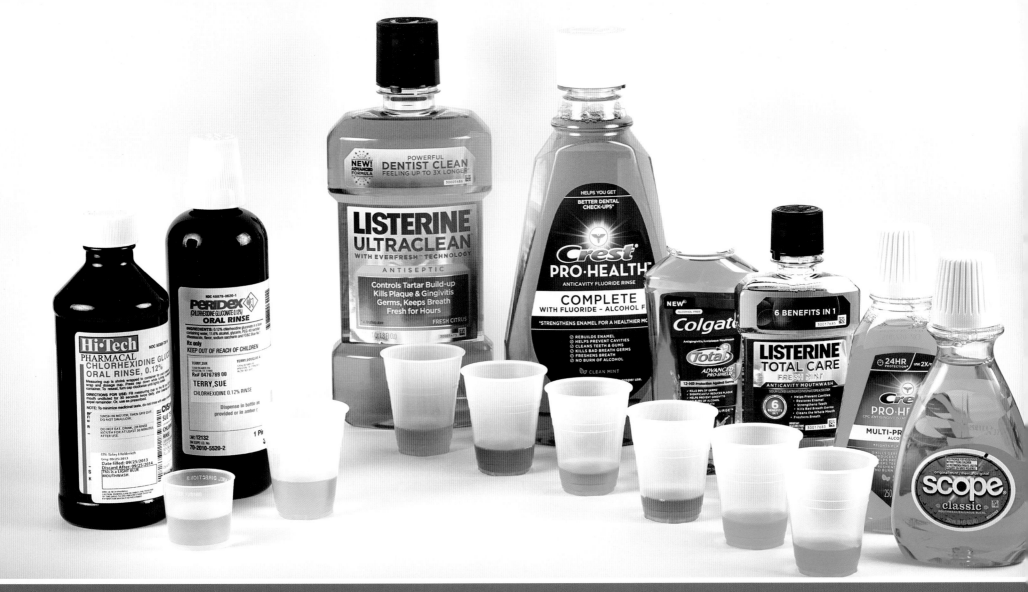

Mechanical cleaning of food and plaque from the mouth by brushing and flossing are limited in their reach, and the simple action of rinsing with mouthwashes provides an effective method for accessing difficult-to-clean areas of the mouth. However, mouthrinses are not a substitute for mechanical oral hygiene techniques. Before using mouthrinses, the teeth should be as clean as possible. When using anticavity rinses, do not rinse, eat, or drink for 30 minutes after use to prevent dilution of the fluoride.

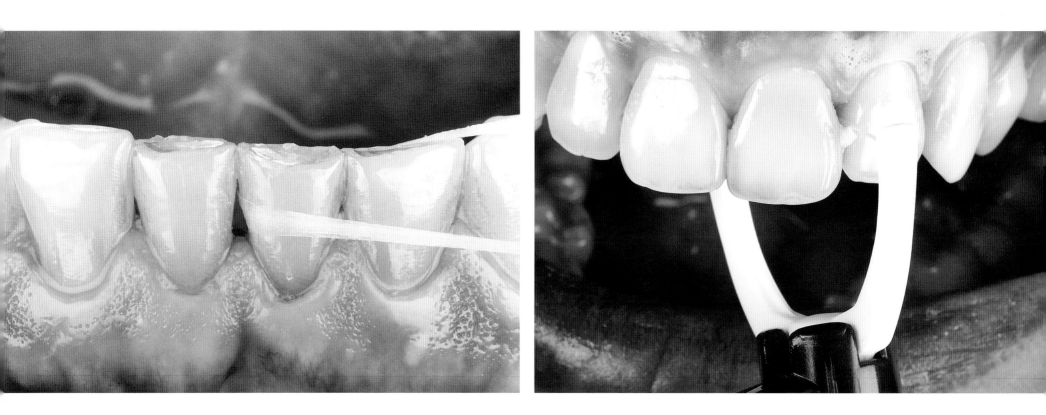

A tooth has five surfaces. If you forget to floss, you only clean three-fifths (or 60%) of your teeth, while two-fifths (or 40%) remain dirty. The plaque in between your teeth is composed of invisible masses of different bacteria that form every 24 hours and cause gum disease and tooth decay. It is important to floss at least once a day.

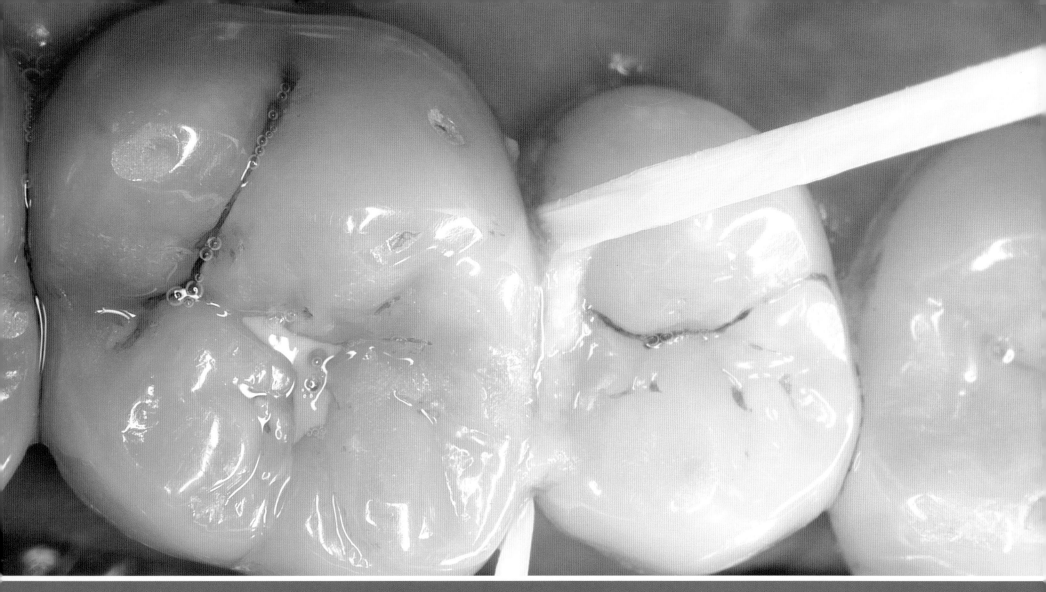

Gently guide the floss between the teeth in a zigzag motion and remember to contour the floss around each tooth surface and move the floss up and down against each tooth surface and under the gum line. Never snap or force the floss, because this may cut or bruise the gum tissue. Don't forget to floss the back side of the last tooth in every arch and along the sides of teeth that border spaces where teeth are missing.

Dental floss comes in a variety of forms: waxed and unwaxed, flavored and unflavored, wide and regular. Waxed floss may be a better choice to use between tight teeth or tight restorations. Also, prethreaded flossers or floss holders can be effective for individuals with limited dexterity.

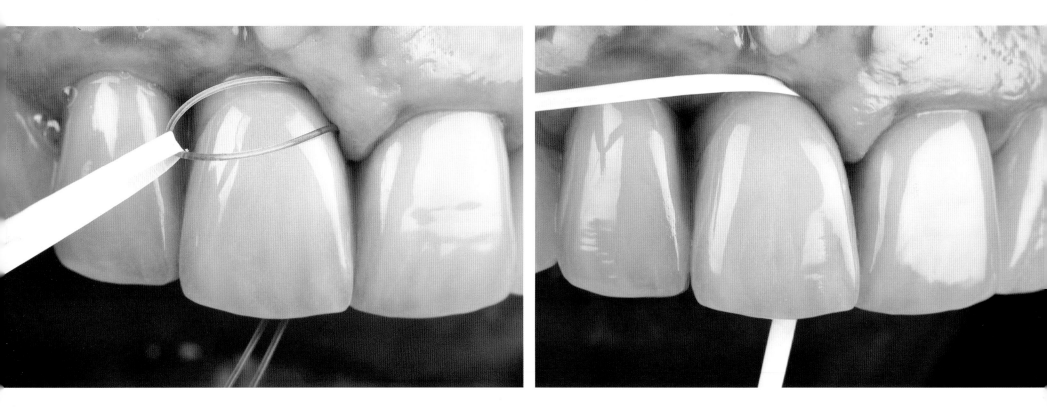

Dental bridge maintenance is important for protecting the teeth supporting the denture from decay, gum disease, and infection. Floss threaders can be used to insert floss under the bridge, allowing the sides of the teeth and the underside of the bridge to be cleaned.

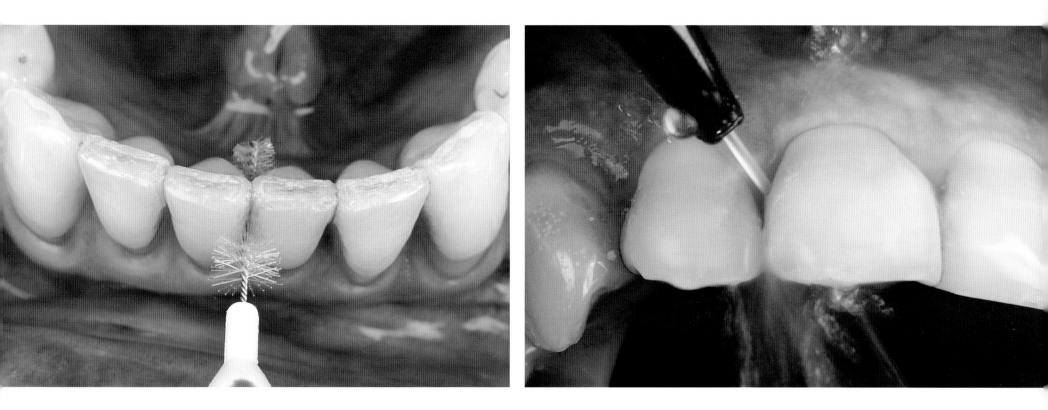

To clean between teeth with larger gaps at the gum line, an interdental brush or proxy brush can be used to remove plaque and debris. These devices are small, slim brushes that have various shapes and sizes to fit into small spaces or gaps in between teeth.

An effective alternative to manual flossing is high-tech flossing with pressurized water and air. These technologies use a combination of water pressure and pulsations (Waterpik) or pressurized air and water microbursts (AirFloss) to remove debris and plaque from the surfaces in between teeth and below the gum line.

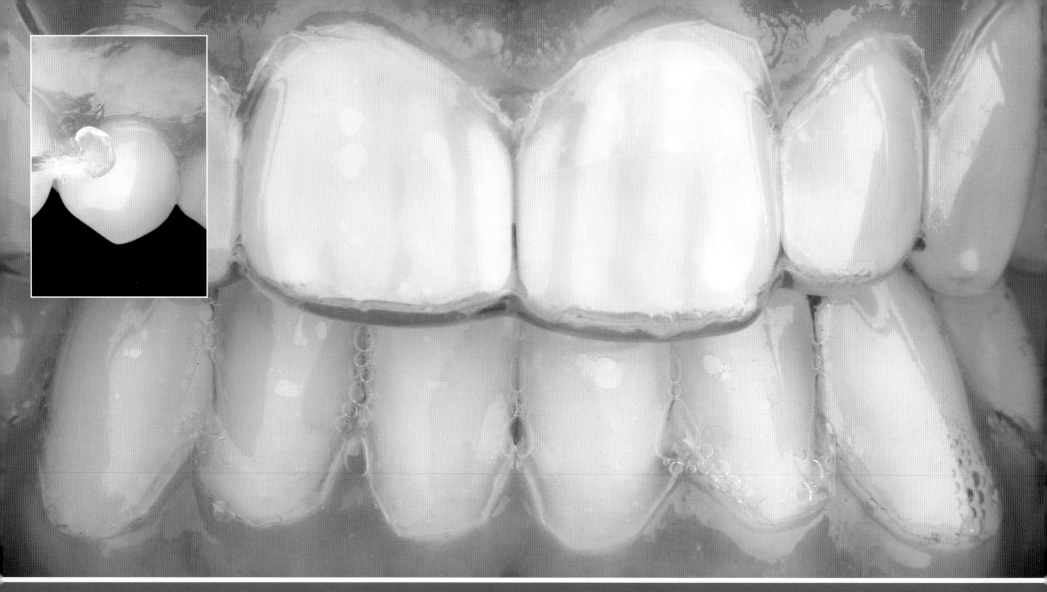

Tooth sensitivity can occur after any tooth-whitening procedure, whether performed at the dental office or at home. The most common tooth-whitening ingredients, hydrogen peroxide and carbamide peroxide, have been known to cause sensitivity as they penetrate the tooth enamel and dentin, which contains extensions to the nerve of the tooth. When peroxide is applied to exposed dentin, it breaks down the *smear layer*, which protects the dentin from oral fluids. Removal of this layer increases cold sensitivity. The peroxide can also irritate the tooth nerve. This irritation or inflammation causes symptoms such as cold sensitivity and a tingling sensation. These side effects usually subside within 1 to 3 days after treatment is discontinued. Individuals with sensitive teeth and gums, receding gums, and/or defective restorations should consult with their dentist before using a tooth-whitening system. Desensitizing products can be applied by your dentist to seal the exposed dentin, and prescribed medication or over-the-counter toothpastes and gels can be used at home before and after the procedure. Also, limiting the consumption of cold beverages and food may reduce and/or eliminate the symptoms.

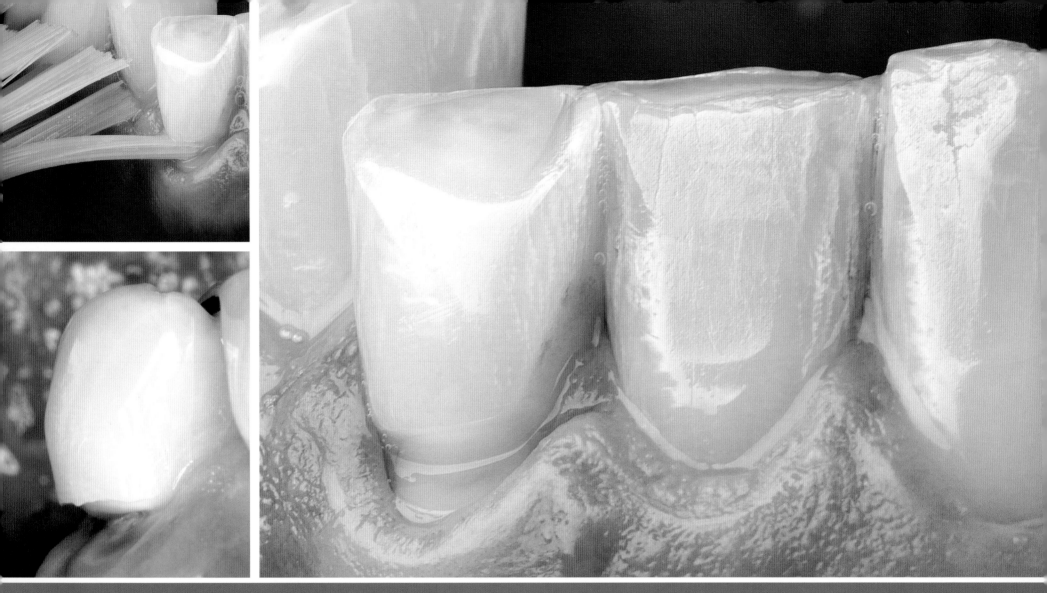

Grooves or notches at the gum line have been referred to as *toothbrush abrasion* and *V-shaped lesions*. This loss of tooth structure at the gum line can be a result of numerous factors such as brushing technique, brushing force, brushing frequency, brushing time, type of brush, diet, abnormal tooth contact, and clenching and grinding. Prevention and management of these gum line defects requires a comprehensive medical and dental history, a thorough clinical examination, and inspection of the way your teeth come together (your bite) by your dentist.

For the large gum line defect shown at left, the patient had no sensitivity but complained of food getting packed in the groove. This defect was the combined result of excessive biting stress on the tooth and improper brushing. A tooth-colored material called *composite* was placed to restore this tooth to its original shape, and the patient was instructed on the proper brushing technique. His bite was also adjusted to eliminate excess forces, and he was given a bite guard to wear at night.

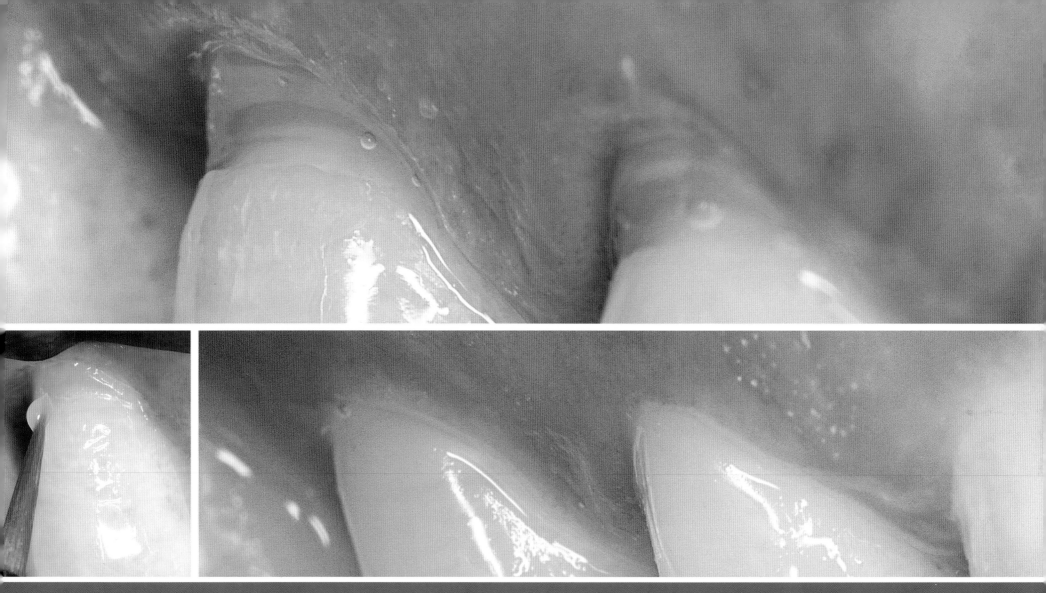

These small notches at the gum line were extremely sensitive. The patient indicated that she drank fruit juices all day long and brushed her teeth rigorously after consumption. Brushing immediately after consumption of acidic foods weakens the tooth and makes it prone to this type of abrasion.

A tooth-colored filling was bonded to the surface, and the pain was eliminated. The patient was advised to regulate her diet and reduce her acidic beverage consumption and to rinse with water after drinking or eating any acidic foods or drinks to neutralize the acids. Also, she was instructed not to brush for at least an hour after any acidic consumption (eg, juice, fruit, soda, coffee, wine).

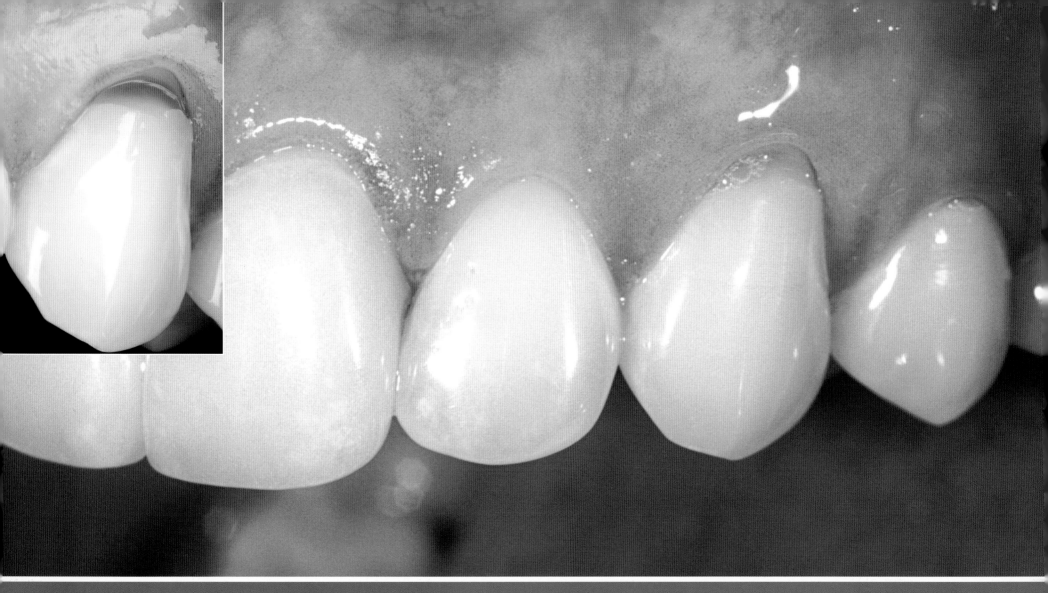

This small V-shaped groove at the gum line was extremely sensitive. The patient indicated that she brushed routinely three to four times a day with a hard-bristle toothbrush and used a smoker's toothpaste. Sometimes these defects are dark yellow in color because the enamel is thin at the neck of the tooth and is easily broken down, exposing the softer dentin (which is dark yellow). The patient had a history of grinding and clenching, which caused wear that was exacerbated by her improper brushing technique. A tooth-colored filling was bonded to replace the enamel surface, and the pain was eliminated. The patient was instructed to use a less abrasive toothpaste and to discontinue smoking and was given a bite guard to wear at night.

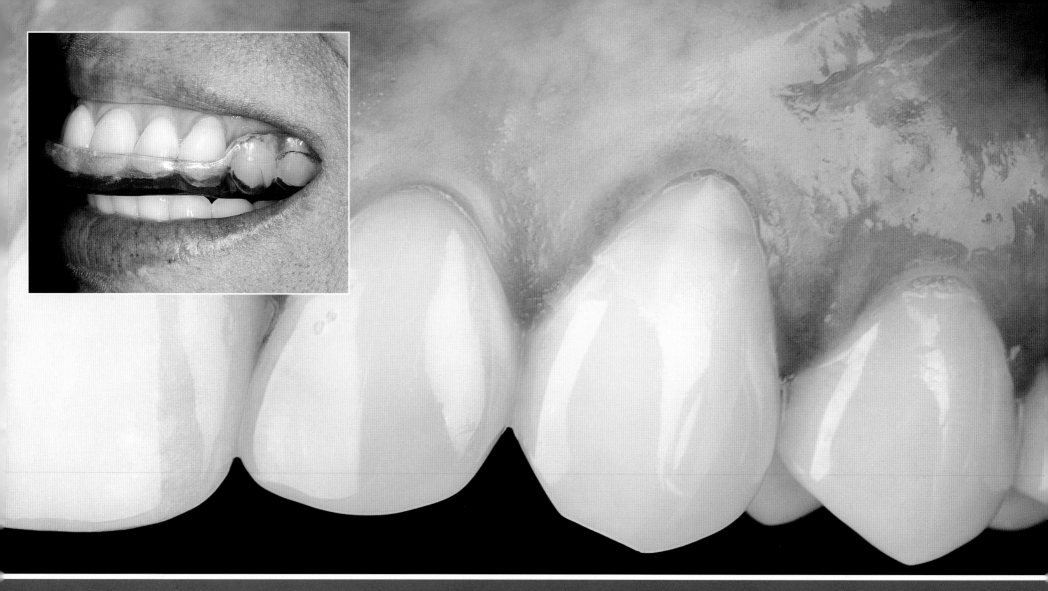

Grinding your teeth can worsen gum line defects and most often occurs during sleep. One management method for nighttime clenching and grinding is to wear a removable bite guard during sleeping hours. These guards limit clenching, prevent surface damage to the teeth, and reduce the possibility of restoration failure (such as a broken crown). In stressful times, your dentist may suggest wearing the guard during waking hours. The splints are made of acrylic and are molded to fit the upper or lower arches of the teeth. An improper fit can cause further damage to your teeth and gums and permanent changes in the bite, so it is important that you seek dental care instead of using an over-the-counter device.

Saliva is a unique biologic fluid. It plays a significant role in maintaining oral health and is nature's primary defense system for the mouth. Healthy saliva neutralizes acid challenges, flushes food and bacteria from the mouth, and acts as a lubricant to wash the teeth. This protective mechanism can be overwhelmed by bacterial action and by strong acids from the stomach and by certain foods. Carbohydrates in particular can make certain bacteria more destructive in dental plaque and create an unhealthy environment that promotes the initiation and progression of tooth decay.

This patient's saliva was unhealthy, and the demineralization process resulted in tooth decay.

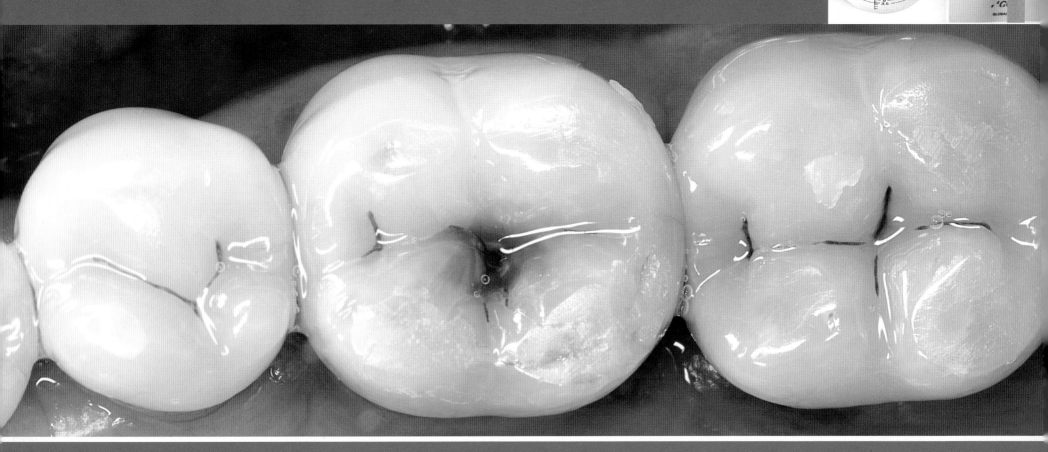

Salivary tests can be used by your dentist to measure and monitor the quality and condition of your saliva. These tests can be used for identifying contributing factors and developing strategies for the prevention and treatment of tooth decay.

This patient's saliva was acid challenged with a pH of 5.5, which indicates an unhealthy environment that facilitates the demineralization process. To combat this deleterious effect, the patient was shown the proper brushing and flossing technique and was advised to regulate diet, increase water intake, and increase salivary stimulation by chewing a sugarless gum or gum containing xylitol.

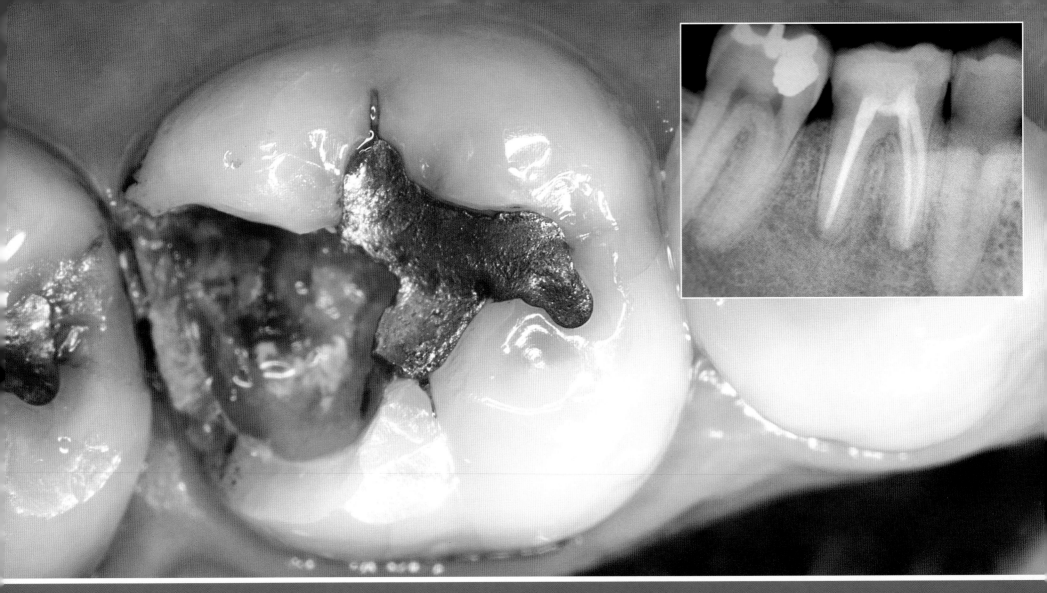

Dental caries, also known as *tooth decay* or a *cavity*, is an infection that is bacterial in origin. You may not be aware of the disease in its early stages. The demineralization process begins as a white spot or a microcavity. As the enamel and dentin are destroyed, the cavity becomes more noticeable.

The tooth in this photograph was weakened by extensive decay, and the tooth fractured during chewing. The patient avoided treatment until a tooth-ache occurred with constant pain. The decay had progressed to the nerve tissue in the center of the tooth, which required root canal treatment. The tooth was restored, and the patient was given dietary modifications, instructed on improved brushing and flossing techniques, and informed of the importance of early detection of tooth decay through routine maintenance visits with a dental professional.

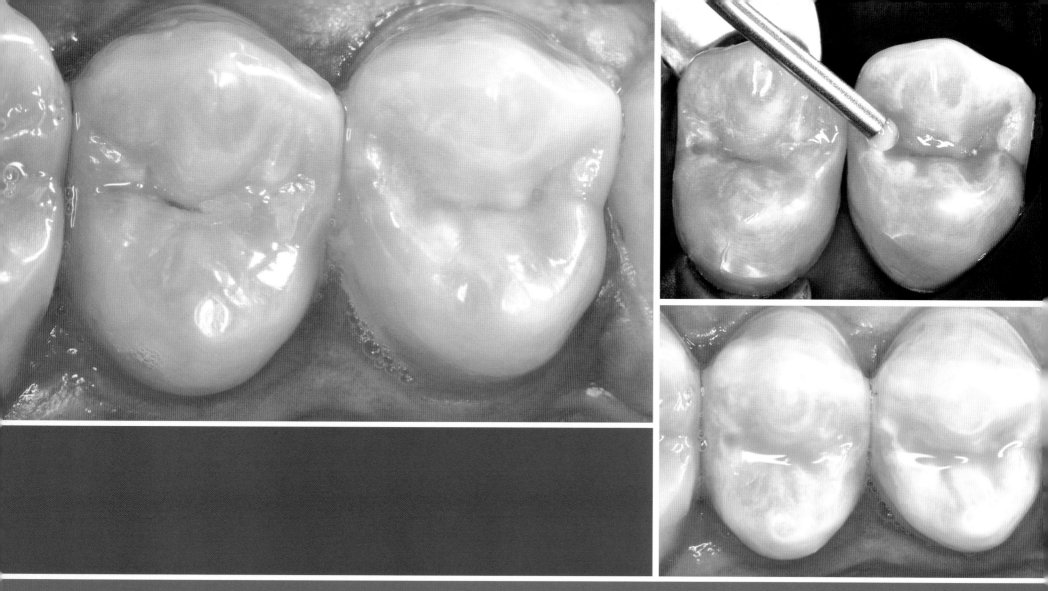

Your back teeth have small grooves and "depressions" called *pits* and *fissures* on their biting surfaces, which can become traps for food and liquid that contain sugar. The sugar can be converted into acid by resident bacteria in plaque and demineralize the tooth surface. Dental sealants are thin, plastic coatings that can be applied to these grooves. This coating protects the chewing surfaces from tooth decay by keeping bacteria and food particles out of the grooves. However, sealants can wear out in time, so they should be checked routinely by a dentist.

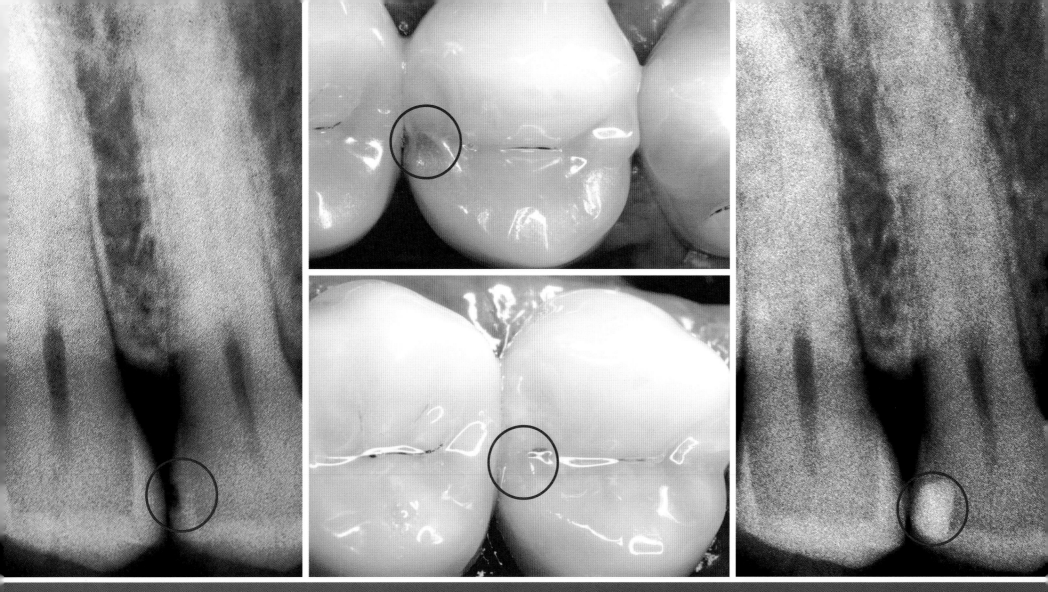

Tooth decay on the surfaces between teeth sometimes cannot be detected by just visual examination of the teeth. An x-ray is required to detect these demineralization areas. Early detection can result in less invasive treatment and sometimes prompt remineralization procedures. This patient's decay was detected after the demineralization process had destroyed the enamel. A small tooth-colored composite filling restored the cavity. Remember, brushing cleans three surfaces of the tooth. This patient brushed his teeth but neglected to floss, leaving two-fifths dirty and resulting in tooth decay between the teeth.

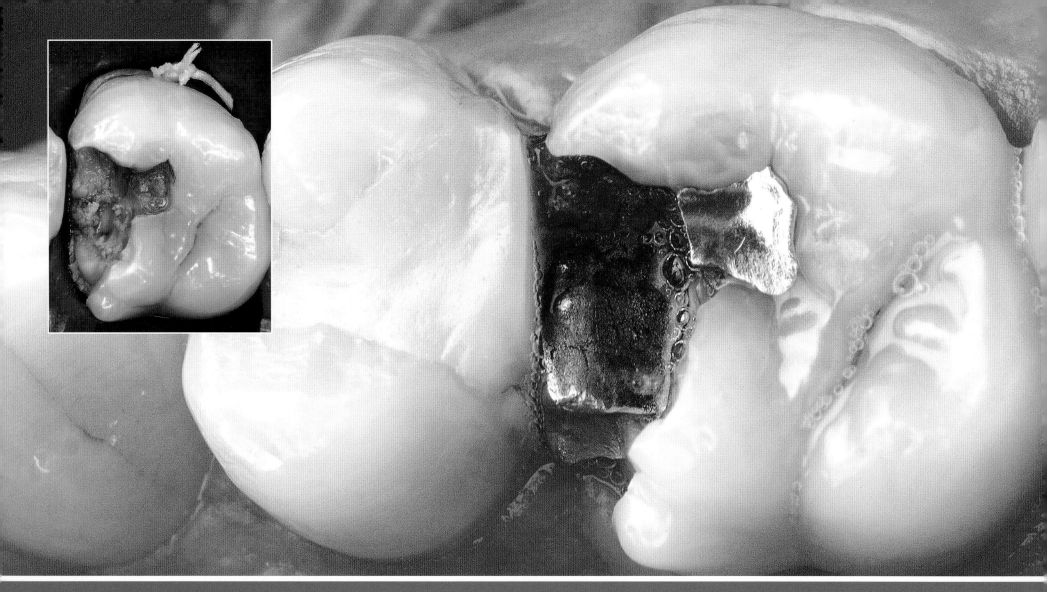

The primary reason for replacing a restoration is recurring tooth decay. Aggressive forms of tooth decay are usually associated with inadequate salivary output or frequent exposure to fermentable carbohydrates.

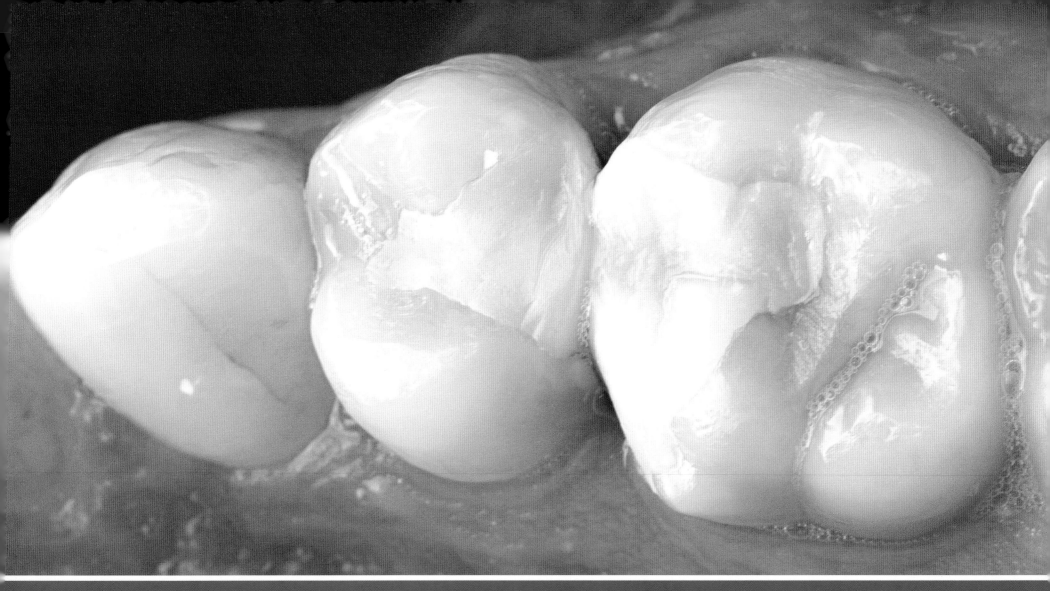

To reduce the potential for tooth decay, a bioactive fluoride-containing filling can be placed in the cavity. This filling can act as a reservoir for the fluoride and thereby continually protect the tooth from decay.

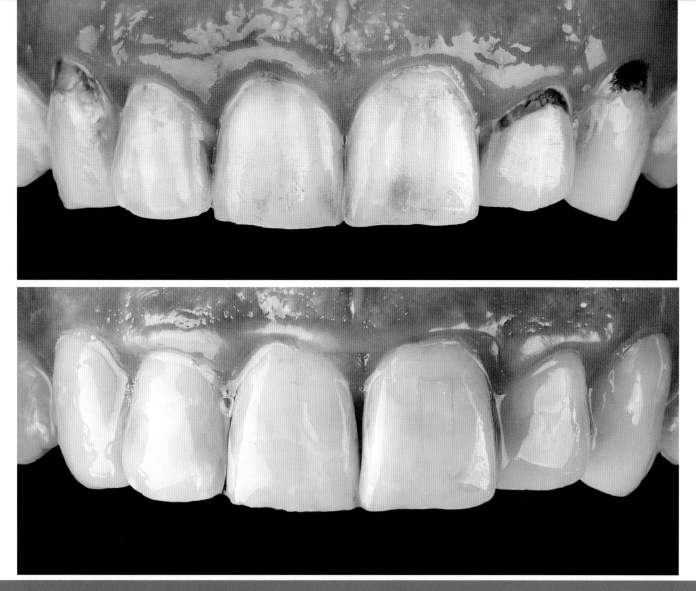

This 38-year-old patient had severe tooth decay from sipping soda throughout the day. Before the teeth were restored with tooth-colored restorations, the patient was instructed to reduce the frequency of his carbohydrate and sugar intake; to use a straw for sugary drinks and to rinse with water after any sugar intake; to use a toothpaste, gel, or rinse containing fluoride alone or in combination with calcium and phosphate; to increase his water intake; and to increase salivary flow by chewing sugarless or xylitol-containing gum. He was also instructed on proper brushing and flossing techniques.

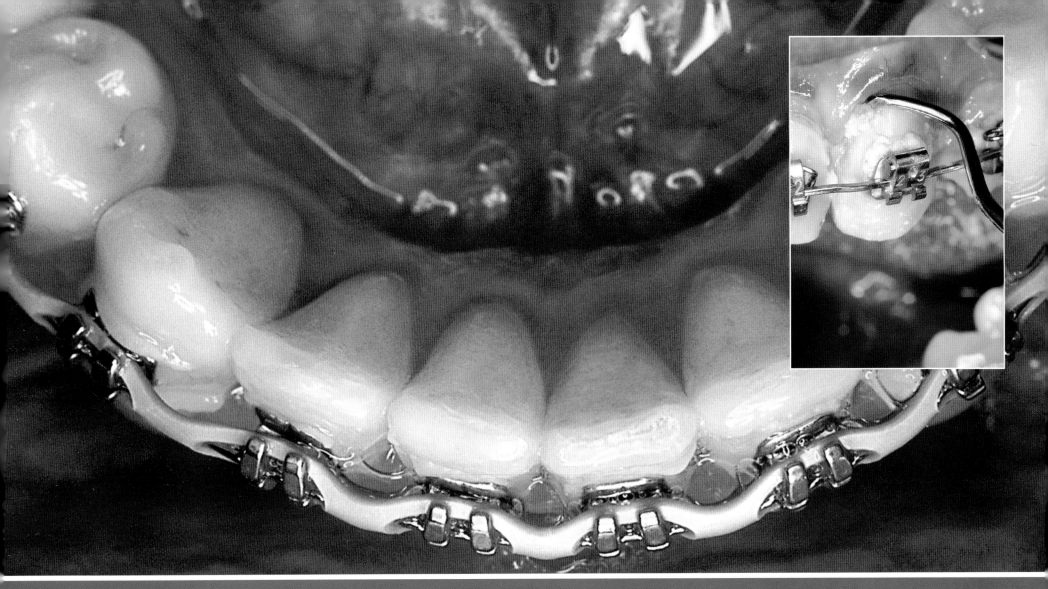

Braces act as a trap for food debris and plaque. White spots of demineralization usually outline the area of the bracket. Sometimes these spots can be sensitive. To prevent plaque accumulation, it is important to brush and floss twice a day and to be monitored by your dentist and orthodontist at routine visits. Also, while wearing braces, another effective way to prevent white spots is to remineralize the teeth with a toothpaste, gel, or rinse containing fluoride alone or in combination with calcium and phosphate.

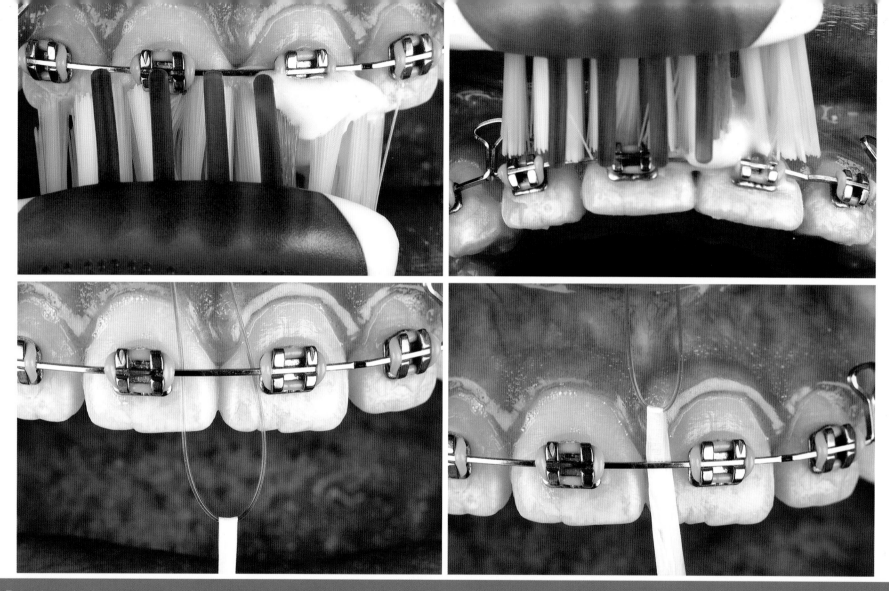

Brushing with braces can be tricky because of all the hardware, but proper brushing and flossing is necessary to prevent cavities and white spots (demineralization) from forming on the teeth around the braces. Follow the regular brushing and flossing technique, but also brush around the brackets and between the braces and wire. It is important to brush after every meal with a soft-bristle brush and fluoridated toothpaste.

Space between the teeth is often unreachable with a regular toothbrush. A floss threader can be used to guide the floss around the braces, in the gum areas, and in between the teeth. Remember to visit your family dentist at regular 6-month visits for proper cleaning and examinations throughout your orthodontic treatment.

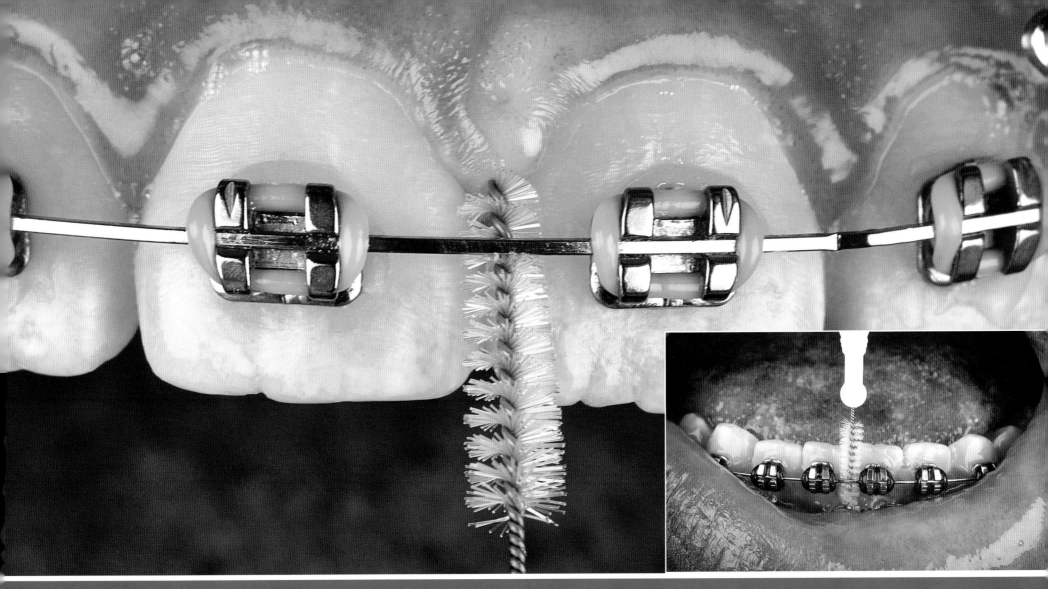

It is difficult to thoroughly clean the surfaces around and between the bonded brackets with a toothbrush. An interdental brush can be useful in maneuvering under orthodontic wires to clean the surface next to the bracket and in between the teeth and remove plaque and food debris. However, be careful not to damage your braces—always use low force and gentle movements.

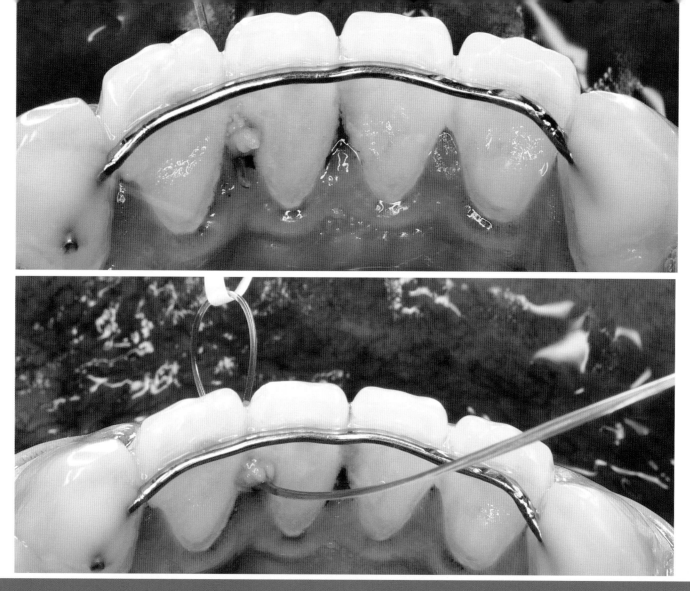

After orthodontic treatment is completed and the braces are removed, a fixed orthodontic wire is often bonded to the teeth to ensure that the position and spacing of the teeth remain the same. Improper care of this wire can result in infected gums. A floss threader can be used to insert and maneuver the floss and clean the surfaces between the teeth. If plaque continues to build up, it can become mineralized to form calculus deposits (tartar) around the wire and the teeth, which can lead to periodontal disease.

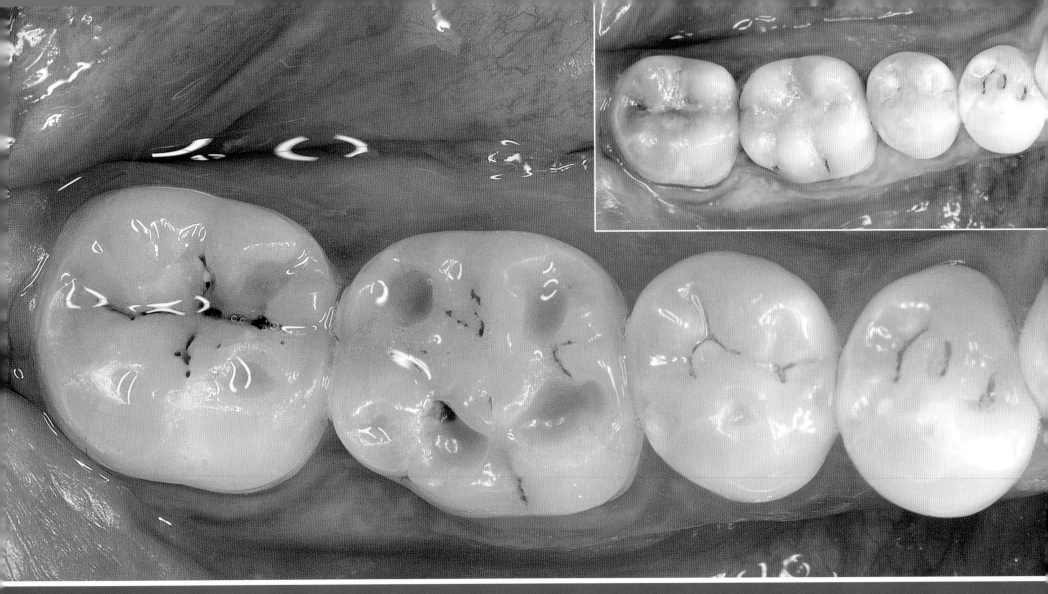

Advanced attritional wear is an increasing challenge as individuals try to retain their natural teeth for their lifetime. *Attrition* is the physical wear of tooth substance or dental restoration caused by tooth contact between the opposing or adjacent tooth surfaces. Functional habits such as chewing are not the main cause of tooth wear. It is the result of abnormal tooth clenching and grinding, called *bruxism*. Bruxism is the most common sleep disorder. For adults, this habit can occur during the day and at night. Bruxism can be caused by stress, anxiety, frustration, competitiveness, abnormal alignment of upper and lower teeth, and other medical conditions. The symptoms can include tooth flattening, cupping, shortening, and chipping; fractured teeth and restorations; sensitivity; restricted jaw movements; chewing of the cheek; creasing in the corners of the mouth; insomnia; earache; headache; jaw pain; prominent jaw muscles; and even loss of teeth. Besides restoring the tooth wear with dental restorations, careful monitoring of the extent and rate of tooth and restoration wear should be part of your routine dental treatment management. Also, to prevent further damage to your teeth, an acrylic bite guard designed for the upper or lower teeth should be worn on a long-term basis during sleep and during stressful episodes.

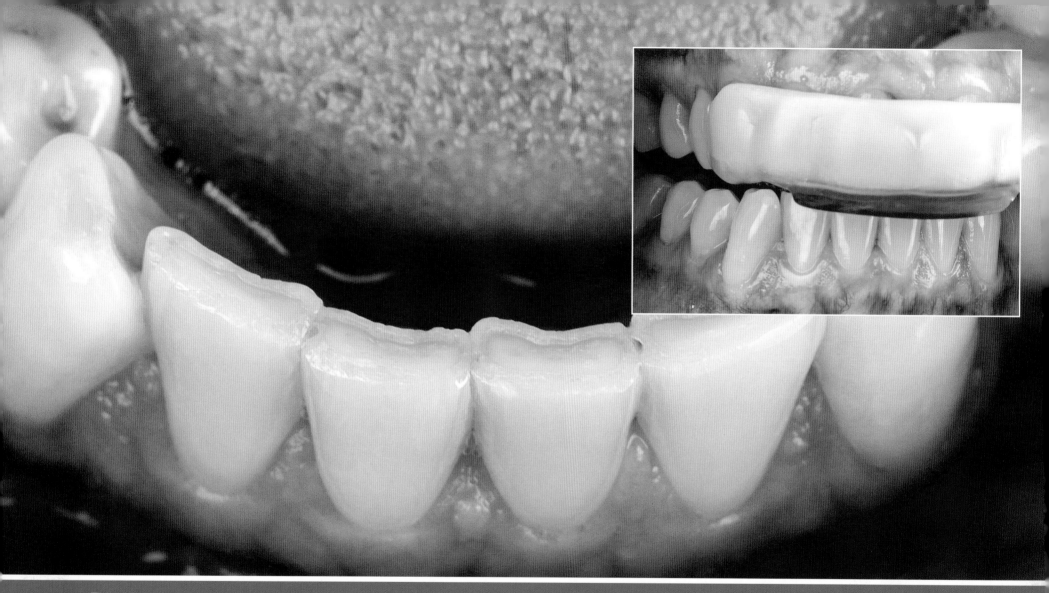

This 45-year-old patient was diagnosed with bruxism but was not aware of the problem because it occurred mainly during sleeping. The patient's husband was interviewed and indicated that her grinding was a nuisance to his sleeping. No restorative treatment was required during this time because of early intervention, but the condition was monitored at future dental visits. Also, to prevent further wear, an acrylic bite guard was designed for her upper teeth to be worn on a long-term basis during sleep and during periods of stress.

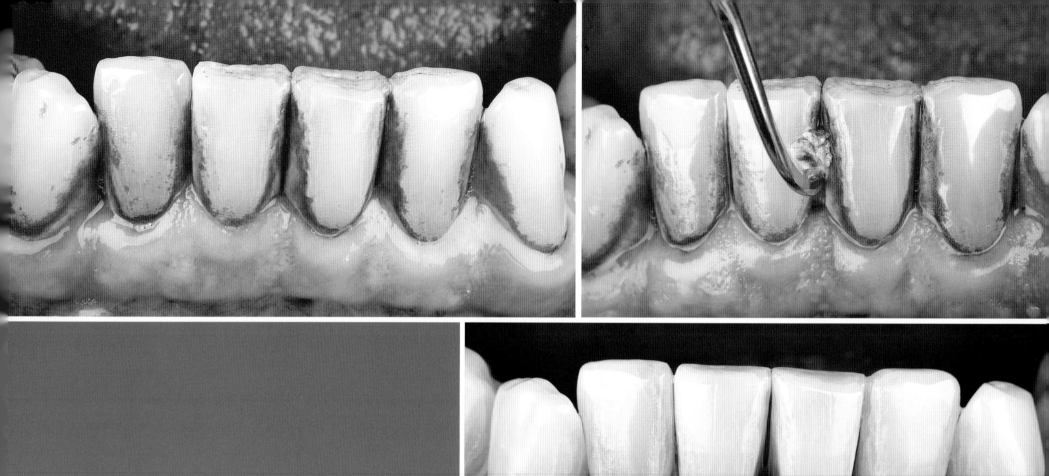

Therapeutic oral rinses containing the ingredient chlorhexidine gluconate are used in the treatment and management of gingivitis. This rinse decreases bacteria in the mouth, reduces redness and swelling of the gums, controls gum bleeding, and protects against gingivitis. It may cause some tooth and restoration discoloration and increase calculus (tartar) formation. Tooth-colored restorations can have permanent discoloration.

To minimize discoloration, you should brush and floss before rinsing and closely brush areas that begin to discolor. Professional cleaning and/or bleaching at the dental office can remove tartar and staining *(bottom photograph)*.

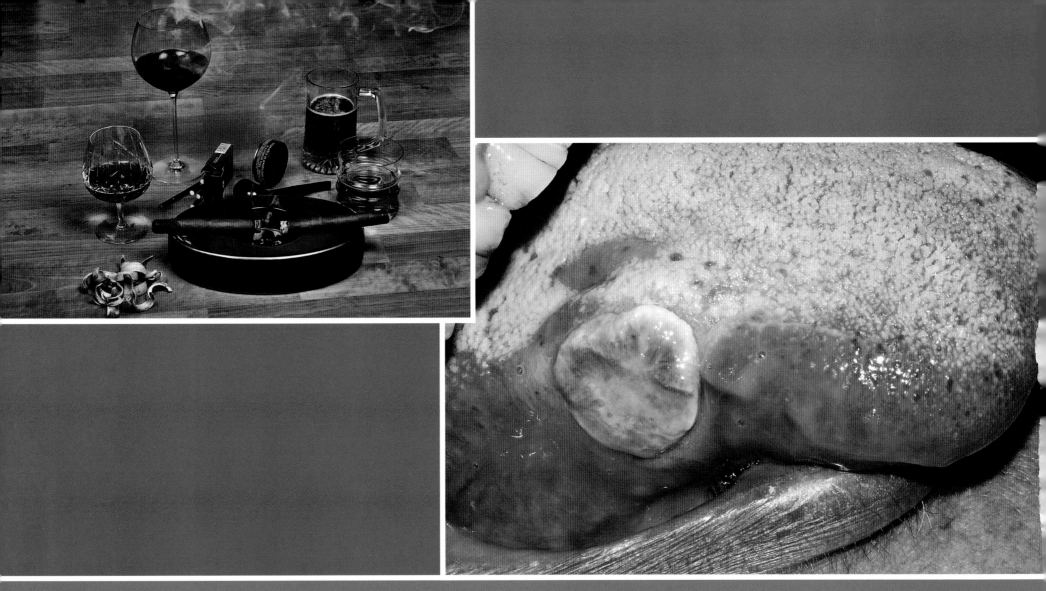

It is well established that tobacco, alone or in combination with alcohol, greatly increases the risk of oral, laryngeal, pharyngeal, and esophageal cancers. In addition, regular chewers of betel quid (chew) and areca nut have a high risk of damaging their gums, scarring the inside of their mouth, and developing cancer of the mouth, pharynx, and esophagus.

This 40-year-old patient was a smoker and visited his dentist for an evaluation of his tongue. He indicated that the growth had been there for weeks and was painful. He was diagnosed with squamous cell carcinoma. Once the lesion has progressed and penetrated adjacent structures, it is referred to as *invasive squamous cell carcinoma*. Once the carcinoma becomes invasive, it is able to spread to other parts of the body, including major organs, and cause a metastasis or secondary tumor to form. You should visit your dentist and/or physician for an evaluation if you have a mouth ulcer that has remained for more than 2 weeks.